KNOWLEDGE GUIDE TO
SCOLIOSIS

Essential Manual To Insights On Diagnosis, Treatment Options, And Pain Relief For Spinal Curvature

DR. AARON BRANUM

Copyright © 2024 BY DR. AARON BRANUM

All rights reserved. Except for brief quotations embodied in critical reviews and certain other noncommercial uses permitted by copyright law, no part of this publication may be reproduced, distributed, or transmitted in any form or by any means, Including photocopying, recording, or other electronic or mechanical methods, without the prior written permission of the publisher.

Disclaimer:

The data in this book, is solely meant to be informative and instructional.

This book is not intended to replace expert medical advice, diagnosis, or care. No medical, health, or other professional services are offered by the author, publisher, or any affiliated parties

Individual outcomes may differ in the practice of these therapies, which entail a variety of approaches and methodologies.

A one-on-one session with a trained or certified healthcare professional is still preferable. It is best to consult a trained healthcare provider before making any decisions regarding your health.

The author of this book is not affiliated with any specific website, product, or organization related to any of these therapies.

All reasonable measures have been taken by the author and publisher to guarantee the authenticity and dependability of the material contained in this book

Contents

- CHAPTER ONE 17
  - THE SPINE'S ANATOMIA: 17
    - The Spine's Structure: 17
    - The Function Of Ligaments, Discs, And Vertebrae 18
    - The Influence Of Spinal Curvature On Posture: 19
    - Spinal Alignment's Significance For General Health 19
    - Typical Spinal Conditions 20
- CHAPTER TWO 23
  - DIAGNOSIS AND EVALUATION 23
    - Scoliosis Symptoms And Indications 23
    - Physical Assessment And Screenings 24
    - Imaging Methods Include CT Scans, Mris, And X-Rays. 25
    - Grading Of Severity: Mild, Moderate, And Severe 26
    - Comprehending Cobb Angle Measurements 27
- CHAPTER THREE 29

OPTIONS FOR SCOLIOSIS TREATMENT 29

Seeing And Keeping An Eye On 29

Bracing: Kinds, Applications, And Efficiency 29

Exercises In Physical Therapy For Scoliosis 31

When Surgical Interventions Are Required 32

Complementary Methods And Alternative Therapies 34

CHAPTER FOUR 37

CONSIDERING SCOLIOSIS 37

Coping Techniques For Pain Control 37

Sustaining Flexibility And Mobility 39

Assistive Devices And Adaptive Equipment 42

Effects On The Mind And Emotional Assistance 44

CHAPTER FIVE 47

LIFESTYLE CHANGES FOR IMPROVED SPINAL HEALTH 47

Pediatric Scoliosis: Prompt Identification And Handling 50

Orthopedic Care For Children 51

Extended Prognosis And Aftercare 52

Resources For Parents And Carers Of Support 53

CHAPTER SIX 55

AVAILABLE IN ADULTS 55

Reasons For Adult-Onset Scoliosis And How It Develops 55

Degenerative Spinal Alterations 57

Techniques For Adult Pain Management ... 58

Surgical Indications And Results.............. 60

Problems With Life Quality And Coping Strategies 62

CHAPTER SEVEN 65

SCOLIOSIS PREVENTION AND MAINTENANCE 65

Awareness Of Posture Is Crucial 65

Stretching And Exercise For A Healthy Spine 66

Ergonomic Guidelines For Typical Tasks ... 67

Dietary Aspects Of Bone Health............... 69

Frequent Exams And Preventive Actions...70
CHAPTER EIGHT...................................73
  A FAQ AND A COMMON ASK: 73
    Could Scoliosis Be Avoided?....................73
    How Might Pregnancy Be Impacted By Scoliosis?...74
    Does Age Cause Scoliosis To Worsen?.......75
    Are There Any Scoliosis Natural Therapies Available? 76

ABOUT THIS BOOK

The "Knowledge Guide to Scoliosis" is an invaluable tool that provides a thorough understanding of scoliosis, a disorder that has a significant influence on people's lives. This book delves into the complex aspects of scoliosis, explaining its various aspects from its definition to its treatment, providing patients and carers with insightful information.

The book begins an educational journey by explaining the basic elements of scoliosis, from its different forms (idiopathic, congenital, and neuromuscular) to debunking common misconceptions and revealing truthful data. By highlighting the importance of early detection, readers are equipped to identify symptoms early on, facilitating prompt action and better results.

In addition, the complex structure of the spine is thoroughly examined, clarifying the functions of ligaments, discs, and vertebrae in preserving spinal integrity. Comprehending the curvature of the spine and how it affects posture highlights the significance of spinal alignment for general health, and providing information on common spinal illnesses helps readers better understand related conditions.

The procedures for diagnosis and assessment are described in great detail, giving readers the knowledge they need to appropriately identify symptoms, grade severity, and navigate signals. The reader is provided with a comprehensive understanding of diagnostic modalities, encompassing physical tests and advanced imaging techniques such as MRI scans and X-rays, as well as the subtle interpretation of Cobb angle measurements.

Regarding therapeutic approaches, the book outlines a variety of techniques, such as bracing and observation, as well as surgical procedures and complementary therapies. The book embraces the complete well-being of people with scoliosis by going beyond medical interventions and providing a thorough discussion of coping mechanisms, maintaining mobility, and psychological support.

Tailored parts address specific issues for both adult and pediatric populations. These issues include long-term prognoses, adult degenerative changes, and early identification in youngsters. In addition, preventative and maintenance
techniques together with informative FAQs provide helpful advice for dealing with day-to-day difficulties and encouraging a proactive attitude to spinal health.

Beyond the traditional bounds of medical literature, "Knowledge Guide to Scoliosis" acts as a guiding light of empowerment for people with scoliosis and their families as they navigate its complicated issues. Its all-encompassing methodology, enhanced by practical observations and empathetic direction, makes it an invaluable ally on the path to comprehending, coping with, and prospering from scoliosis.

Recognition Of Scoliosis

Scoliosis: What Is It?

An abnormal curvature of the spine is a characteristic of the medical condition of scoliosis. The spine may not follow a straight path from the neck to the lower back, but rather a sideways "S" or "C" shape. Depending on its intensity and evolution, this curvature can range from mild to severe and result in a variety of symptoms and consequences.

Scoliosis Types

Unknown Scoliosis

Roughly 80% of scoliosis instances are of the idiopathic variety, which is the most prevalent. It usually appears in adolescence, and its source is unknown. In order to stop future curvature, idiopathic scoliosis may need to be treated or monitored over time.

Origin of Scoliosis

Congenital scoliosis is the result of aberrant prenatal spinal development. It frequently exists from birth or emerges in the early years of life. The degree of this kind of scoliosis varies based on the extent of the deformity and is brought on by anomalies in the creation of the vertebrae.

Scoliosis Neuromuscular

Underlying neurological or muscular disorders including cerebral palsy, muscular dystrophy, or spinal cord injuries are linked to neuromuscular scoliosis. Compared to other forms of scoliosis, neuromuscular scoliosis usually causes more severe and fast curvature of the spine. Treatment for this kind frequently entails treating the underlying musculoskeletal or neurological condition.

The Value of Early Identification

For scoliosis to be managed and treated effectively, early identification is essential. Frequent screenings can assist in detecting spinal curvature early on, particularly throughout adolescence when scoliosis is most likely to develop. Early detection of scoliosis facilitates prompt intervention, thereby halting future curvature progression and reducing the risk of consequences.

Myths vs. Reality Regarding Scoliosis

Myth: Only women are affected by scoliosis.

Factual statement: Although scoliosis is more common in women, it can afflict individuals of any gender.

Myth: Back discomfort is always a result of scoliosis.

Truth: Back discomfort is not a common symptom of scoliosis. While it is not always there, pain can happen in certain situations.

Myth: Exercise is the only way to treat scoliosis.

Factual statement: Although physical therapy and exercise can assist control of scoliosis and enhance muscular strength and flexibility, they are unable to correct the underlying curvature of the spine.

Scoliosis's Effects on Everyday Life

Scoliosis can make daily living difficult in a number of ways. People with scoliosis may encounter the following symptoms, contingent on the degree of the spine curvature and related conditions:

Physical limitations: Prolonged sitting, standing, or walking can be uncomfortable for people with severe scoliosis due to movement restrictions.

Impact on emotions: In particular, scoliosis in adolescents may have an impact on body image and self-esteem. Managing a visible curvature of the spine may cause social anxiety and feelings of self-consciousness.

Medical management: Bracing, physical therapy, frequent medical visits, and, in certain situations, surgery, can all be used to treat scoliosis. Daily schedules may be impacted, and changes may be necessary to meet treatment requirements.

People can better manage the difficulties posed by scoliosis and look for the right support and treatment choices if they are aware of how the condition affects their day-to-day functioning. Preventive care and early identification are essential for reducing the negative effects of scoliosis on general health.

CHAPTER ONE

THE SPINE'S ANATOMIA:

The Spine's Structure:

With 33 vertebrae piled on top of one another to form a flexible and supporting column, the spine is an amazing structure.

The areas of these vertebrae include sacral, coccygeal, lumbar (lower back), thoracic (mid-back), and cervical (neck).

There are seven vertebrae in the cervical spine, twelve in the thoracic spine, five in the lumbar spine, and five vertebrae combined in the sacral and coccygeal areas.

An intervertebral disc, which acts as a cushion and gives the spine flexibility, is located between each vertebra.

The annulus fibrosus, a strong outer layer, and the nucleus pulposus, an inner core that resembles gel, make up these discs.

The Function Of Ligaments, Discs, And Vertebrae

The vertebrae are the building blocks of the spine; they protect and stabilize the spinal cord.

The processes, which are bony protrusions on each vertebra, act as attachment places for muscles and ligaments, providing stability and mobility.

By absorbing pressure and shock, intervertebral discs help keep the vertebrae from rubbing against one another when moving. The strong bands of connective tissue called ligaments stabilize the spine by holding the vertebrae together.

The Influence Of Spinal Curvature On Posture:

From a side perspective, the naturally curved spine forms a S shape. These curves aid in maintaining balance and distributing the body's weight equally. Scoliosis, kyphosis, and lordosis are examples of spinal curvature problems that can result from anomalies in these curves.

The characteristic of scoliosis is a sideways curvature of the spine, which can cause the spine to rotate and cause uneven shoulder or hip height. This may result in discomfort and posture imbalances, which could harm one's looks and self-esteem.

Spinal Alignment's Significance For General Health

It is essential to maintain appropriate spinal alignment for general health and well-being.

Proper alignment of the spine facilitates smooth movement, lessens strain on muscles and ligaments, and aids in supporting the weight of the body.

In addition to reducing pain and dysfunction, proper spinal alignment makes sure that the nerves leaving the spinal cord are not pinched or inflamed.

Typical Spinal Conditions

A number of prevalent spinal conditions can impact individuals of any age. One of the most common, particularly in teenagers, is scoliosis, which can have mild to severe forms.

Other common spinal abnormalities include lordosis, which involves an excessive inward curvature of the lower back, and kyphosis, which is characterized by an excessively forward rounding of the upper back.

Spinal stenosis, degenerative disc disease, and herniated discs are other common conditions that can result in pain, stiffness, and restricted movement.

In order to manage these spinal illnesses and enhance quality of life, a proper diagnosis and treatment plan are important.

CHAPTER TWO

DIAGNOSIS AND EVALUATION

Scoliosis Symptoms And Indications

Early detection of scoliosis is essential for successful treatment. Depending on the kind and severity of scoliosis, there may be different signs and symptoms.

Asymmetry in the hips, waist, or shoulders is among the most typical signs. Another clue may be a prominent curvature of the spine, particularly while leaning forward.

Sometimes there may be an uneven rib cage or one shoulder blade that protrudes more than the other.

A change in the body's center of gravity or uneven leg lengths are further signs of scoliosis. Furthermore, respiratory difficulties, muscular exhaustion, and back discomfort are possible side effects of scoliosis.

Physical Assessment And Screenings

Accurate diagnosis of scoliosis requires a thorough physical examination. Healthcare practitioners may evaluate a patient's posture, gait, and range of motion during a physical examination.

They could also take a measurement of the legs' length to look for any differences. To find any anomalies or asymmetries, palpate the spine and the muscles around it.

Furthermore, early detection of spine curvature can be facilitated by a variety of screening techniques, including the Adam's Forward Bend Test and scoliometer readings.

In order to detect scoliosis in children and adolescents, these screenings are frequently carried out in schools or during standard physical examinations.

Imaging Methods Include CT Scans, Mris, And X-Rays.

Imaging methods are vital for confirming a diagnosis of scoliosis and assessing its severity. The main imaging method for determining the curvature and alignment of the spine is X-rays.

They give precise measurements of the degree of curvature by providing comprehensive images of the spine from various perspectives, which are useful to healthcare practitioners.

To further assess spinal problems, computed tomography (CT) and magnetic resonance imaging (MRI) scans may be advised in specific circumstances.

While CT scans offer precise images of the bones and joints, MRI scans are especially helpful for evaluating soft tissues, such as discs and nerves.

Grading Of Severity: Mild, Moderate, And Severe

Following a diagnosis of scoliosis, medical experts categorize the degree of spine curvature using severity grading systems.

This categorization aids in choosing the best course of action for therapy and tracking the condition's evolution over time.

Usually, scoliosis severity is classified as mild, moderate, or severe depending on the curvature's degree, which is expressed in degrees. Less than 20 degrees is considered mild scoliosis, 20 to 50 degrees is considered intermediate scoliosis, and more than 50 degrees is considered severe scoliosis.

Planning a customized course of treatment and managing scoliosis requires an understanding of its severity.

Comprehending Cobb Angle Measurements

The conventional technique for estimating the degree of spine curvature in scoliosis is the Cobb angle measurement.

Drawing lines parallel to the endplates of the curve's most twisted vertebrae allows one to calculate it. The degree of curvature is indicated by the angle created when these lines connect.

Measuring the Cobb angle is essential for determining the degree of scoliosis and tracking its evolution over time.

This assessment is used by medical practitioners to inform treatment choices and assess the efficacy of interventions.

Patients and carers can take an active role in their treatment and make educated decisions about their care when they are aware of Cobb angle measurements.

CHAPTER THREE

OPTIONS FOR SCOLIOSIS TREATMENT

Seeing And Keeping An Eye On

Monitoring and surveillance are essential in the treatment of scoliosis, particularly in mild to moderate cases of the curvature of the spine. It's crucial to see a doctor on a regular basis, usually every four to six months, to monitor the condition's development. Your doctor may use imaging tests, such as X-rays, in addition to physical examinations to determine the degree of curvature at these sessions.

Bracing: Kinds, Applications, And Efficiency

For people with mild scoliosis, bracing is frequently advised, especially throughout growing stages like adolescence. There are several different kinds of braces that are available, such as the Charleston bending brace, Milwaukee brace, and Boston brace. The location and degree of the spinal curvature determine what kind of brace is given.

Bracing is primarily used to apply corrective pressure to the spine in order to stop the curvature from continuing to progress. Braces are normally worn for a set amount of hours every day, mostly while sleeping or not moving around.

The efficacy of the brace depends on wearer compliance, and frequent follow-up visits with the orthopedic specialist are required to track improvement and adjust the brace as needed.

According to studies, bracing can effectively stop or slow down the course of scoliosis, especially if treatment is started when the skeleton is still growing. The degree of curvature, the patient's age, and the patient's compliance with the treatment plan are some of the variables that can affect how well bracing works.

Exercises In Physical Therapy For Scoliosis

Exercises from physical therapy are a vital aspect of the treatment of scoliosis, especially for those with mild to moderate curvature of the spine. By strengthening muscles, enhancing flexibility, and correcting posture, these activities can reduce pain and stop the curvature from getting worse.

A licensed physical therapist will create a customized exercise plan depending on the demands of the client and the degree of their scoliosis. These workouts could involve body awareness and breathing exercises, as well as strengthening, stretching, and core stabilization activities.

Physical therapy for scoliosis requires a commitment to consistency and effort. To get the best effects, it's imperative to consistently and accurately do the exercises as directed. Sustaining proper posture and implementing ergonomic practices into everyday tasks can also enhance the efficiency of physical therapy in the management of scoliosis.

When Surgical Interventions Are Required

Surgical intervention may be advised in cases of severe scoliosis or when alternative treatment methods have failed to stop the curvature's progression. Correction of the spinal deformity and stabilization of the spine to stop future advancement are the main objectives of scoliosis surgery.

Spinal fusion, which joins the vertebrae together using bone grafts and instruments like rods, screws, and hooks, is the standard surgical procedure for scoliosis. This aids in straightening the spine and keeps it from bending much further. The location and degree of the curvature, as well as the patient's general health and lifestyle, will all influence the precise surgical strategy and methods employed.

Scoliosis surgery is regarded as a big treatment, thus it should only be undertaken after considerable thought and consultation with a group of qualified medical experts. Although many scoliosis sufferers find their quality of life improved and their spine curvature properly corrected, surgery is not without danger and necessitates a lengthy recovery period.

Complementary Methods And Alternative Therapies

Some people with scoliosis may look into complementary and alternative therapies in addition to traditional medical treatments in order to manage their condition.

These might include, among other things, Pilates, yoga, acupuncture, and chiropractic care.

Although some people may experience symptom alleviation and an improvement in general well-being from these alternative therapies, it's important to approach them cautiously and with skepticism.

Many alternative treatments for scoliosis are not well-supported by science, and some may even increase the risk of side effects or aggravate the illness if not used correctly.

Consult a healthcare provider, ideally one with experience treating spine disorders, before attempting any complementary or alternative therapy for scoliosis.

They can offer advice on suitable and safe solutions and assist in incorporating them into a thorough treatment plan that is customized to the needs and preferences of the patient.

CHAPTER FOUR

CONSIDERING SCOLIOSIS

Coping Techniques For Pain Control

Living with scoliosis can be difficult, especially when it comes to controlling the pain that comes with the disorder.

Nonetheless, people can enhance their quality of life and reduce suffering by using a variety of coping mechanisms.

Physical therapy combined with regular exercise is one successful strategy. Exercises aimed at building up the surrounding muscles of the spine can alleviate tension and offer support to the afflicted areas.

Stretching exercises can also help reduce stiffness, which frequently aggravates discomfort, and increase flexibility.

Adopting proper posture is another useful tactic. By keeping your posture correct, you can lessen discomfort and pressure on your affected sections of the spine by distributing your weight evenly over it.

Maintaining proper posture during the day can also be facilitated by using supporting pillows and ergonomic furniture.

Additionally, practicing relaxation methods like yoga, meditation, or deep breathing can assist ease body tension and stress, which can worsen scoliosis discomfort.

These methods support mental health in addition to encouraging physical relaxation.

To relieve more severe agony, over-the-counter painkillers or prescribed pain management measures could be required in certain situations.

A healthcare professional's advice is crucial in order to decide on the best course of action depending on each patient's unique needs and the severity of their symptoms.

People with scoliosis who use these coping mechanisms in their daily lives can better control their discomfort and feel better overall.

Sustaining Flexibility And Mobility

For people with scoliosis, maintaining flexibility and mobility is essential to improving their overall physical function and quality of life. The following useful tips can assist in maintaining flexibility and mobility:

For those with scoliosis to improve their mobility and flexibility, regular exercise is crucial.

Stretching, weight training, and aerobic workouts together can assist increase range of motion and decrease stiffness in the surrounding muscles and spine.

Stretching activities that target the muscles impacted by scoliosis particularly can help reduce stress and increase the range of motion.

To improve posture and spinal alignment, pay special attention to stretches that work the hamstrings, back, hips, and chest.

Including low-impact exercises like walking, cycling, or swimming in your routine will assist enhance your general mobility and cardiovascular health without placing undue strain on your spine.

Furthermore, engaging in balance and coordination-enhancing exercises like tai chi or yoga can enhance proprioception and stability, lowering the chance of accidents and falls.

It's crucial to pay attention to your body and refrain from overdoing it, especially if exercising causes you pain or suffering.

To safely develop your strength and flexibility, gradually increase the duration and intensity of your workouts.

By implementing these techniques into your everyday routine, you may preserve your flexibility and range of motion, which will keep you active and involved in the activities you enjoy.

Assistive Devices And Adaptive Equipment

To increase comfort, mobility, and independence while living with scoliosis, assistive devices, and adapted equipment may be needed. The following typical tools can help people with scoliosis in their day-to-day activities:

Orthopedic braces: In order to stop the spine curvature from getting worse, bracing may be advised for those with mild to severe scoliosis. These braces are made in order to suit each person precisely, with the goal of stabilizing and supporting the spine.

Ergonomic furniture: When sitting or working for lengthy periods of time, using ergonomic chairs, desks, and other furniture can assist in encouraging good posture and lessen the strain on the spine.

Assistive devices for daily living: Equipment like reachers, dressing aids, and adaptive utensils can make daily tasks easier for people with scoliosis and lessen the strain on their back and surrounding muscles.

Mobility aids: Canes, walkers, and wheelchairs are examples of devices that can support and assist people who are limited in their ability to move owing to pain or weakness caused by scoliosis.

Tailored cushions and pillows: For people with scoliosis, using cushions and pillows that support optimal spine alignment can help reduce discomfort and improve sleep quality.

The best adaptive technology and assistive gadgets should be chosen in consultation with a healthcare provider or occupational therapist depending on each person's needs and functional skills.

People with scoliosis can increase their comfort, mobility, and independence by using these items in their daily lives, which will improve their overall quality of life.

Effects On The Mind And Emotional Assistance

People who have scoliosis may experience severe psychological effects that impair their quality of life and emotional health. It's critical to address the psychological effects of scoliosis and, if necessary, seek out emotional help. The following are some methods for addressing the psychological effects of scoliosis:

A sense of comprehension, empathy, and connection can be given to those with scoliosis by asking for help from friends, family, or a support group.

It can be quite helpful to share coping mechanisms and experiences with those who are going through comparable difficulties.

Individuals can enhance their general emotional well-being, develop coping mechanisms, and explore and process their feelings connected to scoliosis by participating in talk therapy or counseling with a mental health expert.

Anxiety and tension related to scoliosis can be managed by practicing mindfulness and stress-reduction methods such as progressive muscle relaxation, deep breathing, and meditation.

People who have scoliosis can develop resilience and adaptation in the face of adversity by keeping an optimistic attitude and emphasizing their skills and abilities.

Gaining knowledge about scoliosis and available treatments can enable people to actively manage their condition and speak up for what they need.

Prioritizing self-care and participating in activities that enhance mental and emotional well-being, such as hobbies, exercise, and quality time with loved ones, is crucial for those with scoliosis.

People with scoliosis can improve their overall quality of life and resilience in managing the illness by addressing the psychological effects of the condition and obtaining emotional help when necessary.

CHAPTER FIVE

LIFESTYLE CHANGES FOR IMPROVED SPINAL HEALTH

Changing one's lifestyle can be extremely important for controlling scoliosis symptoms and encouraging improved spine health. The following are some doable methods for implementing lifestyle changes in day-to-day activities:

Keep a healthy weight: Being overweight can aggravate scoliosis symptoms and put additional strain on the spine. Maintaining a healthy weight and lowering the risk of problems can be achieved by following a balanced diet and getting frequent exercise.

Maintain proper posture: Maintaining proper posture can assist reduce pressure on the spine and improve spinal alignment. Pay attention to maintaining a neutral spine alignment, chin tucked, and shoulders back while sitting and standing.

Steer clear of extended sitting or standing: Reducing the amount of time spent sitting or standing up can assist relieve pressure on the spine and avoid pain and stiffness. Take regular breaks to move around, stretch, or switch positions to help release tension and encourage circulation.

Employ good body mechanics: To prevent injuries to the spine, utilize good body mechanics when lifting heavy things or carrying out bending or twisting chores. When it is feasible, avoid twisting actions, bend at the knees, and maintain a straight back.

Purchase supportive footwear: Proper spinal alignment can be promoted and tension on the back and lower extremities can be minimized by wearing supportive footwear with appropriate arch support.

Keep yourself hydrated: Sustaining the body's natural healing processes and preserving spinal health depends on consuming a sufficient amount of water each day.

Prioritize sleep quality: Getting enough restorative sleep is vital for general health and well-being, including spinal health. Make an investment in pillows and a supportive mattress to support healthy spinal alignment and promote sound sleep.

People with scoliosis can enhance their overall quality of life, lessen discomfort, and promote better spinal health by adopting these lifestyle changes into daily activities.

Pediatric Scoliosis: Prompt Identification And Handling

Recognizing Childhood and Adolescent Early Detection

The term "pediatric scoliosis" describes the abnormal curvature of the spine that affects kids and teenagers.

Effective management of this illness requires early identification. Parents need to be on the lookout for symptoms including lopsided shoulders, a protruding shoulder blade, or an uneven waist.

Early identification might be aided by routine screenings performed during pediatric examinations.

Identifying Risk Factors and Growth Patterns

It's critical to comprehend growth patterns when evaluating pediatric scoliosis. Fast growth spurts can make curvature worse, particularly in adolescence.

In addition, scoliosis in children might be predisposed by specific risk factors such as genetics, neuromuscular disorders, or congenital anomalies. Keeping an eye on these variables can help with early action.

Orthopedic Care For Children

Orthopedic care for children is essential to the management of scoliosis. Surgical intervention, bracing, or observation are among the techniques used by orthopedic professionals, depending on the degree and course of the curvature. In order to stop moderate curvature from getting worse, bracing is frequently advised; in severe situations, surgery can be required.

Extended Prognosis And Aftercare

Monitoring the curvature of the spine and scheduling many follow-up sessions are necessary to determine the long-term prognosis of pediatric scoliosis.

Certain situations might be resolved with conservative treatment, while others might need continuous care until adulthood.

Pediatricians and orthopedic specialists work closely together to guarantee prompt treatments and thorough care.

Resources For Parents And Carers Of Support

Parental and carer scoliosis navigation can be challenging. Thankfully, there are lots of support services accessible to offer direction and help.

Educational resources, internet discussion boards, and support groups provide insightful knowledge and emotional support.

Making connections with other families going through comparable difficulties can also help parents feel less alone and more capable of effectively managing their child's illness.

CHAPTER SIX

AVAILABLE IN ADULTS

Reasons For Adult-Onset Scoliosis And How It Develops

Unlike adolescent scoliosis, which normally develops during growth spurts, adult-onset scoliosis develops later in life, usually after the age of 18.

The advancement of a pre-existing curvature that wasn't identified or addressed throughout adolescence is one frequent reason. Degenerative changes in the spine, such as osteoarthritis, vertebral fractures, or disc degeneration, are other causes.

Natural wear and tear on the spine as we age might result in degenerative changes. The spine may become curved as a result of these alterations causing the vertebrae to move out of alignment. Adult onset scoliosis can also be accelerated by the development of muscular weakness and imbalances.

The course of scoliosis that develops in adults differs from person to person. Some people may observe a more fast deterioration of their curvature, while others may see a slow and gradual decline. There are several factors that can affect the rate of advancement, including genetics, lifestyle, and general health.

Adults with scoliosis should keep a close eye on their condition since early discovery and treatment can lessen symptoms and stop further progression. Frequent visits to a medical specialist, such as a physical therapist or orthopedic surgeon, can assist patients in efficiently managing their illness.

Degenerative Spinal Alterations

One of the most prominent contributing factors to adult-onset scoliosis is degenerative changes in the spine.

Disc degeneration is the result of these alterations brought on by the intervertebral discs losing their flexibility and moisture. Consequently, the discs can protrude or rupture, applying pressure to the spinal nerves and producing agony.

Moreover, osteoarthritis, a degenerative joint disease, can impact the spine's facet joints, resulting in stiffness and irritation. Adult scoliosis may develop or worsen as a result of the deterioration of these joints over time.

Adult-onset scoliosis can also be caused by vertebral fractures in addition to osteoarthritis and disc degeneration. The spine may become curved as a result of osteoporosis or trauma-related fractures that change the spine's alignment.

Developing successful treatment plans for scoliosis that develops in adults requires a thorough understanding of the degenerative changes that occur in the spine. Physicians can assist relieve discomfort and stop the curvature from getting worse by treating the underlying degenerative processes.

Techniques For Adult Pain Management

Since many people with adult-onset scoliosis endure persistent back pain as a result of their condition, pain management is an important part of treatment. Thankfully, there are numerous approaches that can be used to reduce pain and enhance quality of life.

For people with scoliosis, physical treatment is frequently advised in order to strengthen the muscles that support the spine and enhance posture. Physical therapists can help reduce pain and increase mobility with certain exercises and stretches.

Medication may be used in addition to physical therapy to treat scoliosis-related pain and inflammation. Ibuprofen and naproxen, two nonsteroidal anti-inflammatory medicines (NSAIDs), can help lessen discomfort and swelling in the affected area.

Injections such as corticosteroids or nerve blocks may be suggested for people with severe or chronic pain in order to temporarily relieve symptoms. These injections assist lessen discomfort and inflammation by focusing on particular pain regions.

Additionally, for certain scoliosis sufferers, complementary therapies like massage therapy, chiropractic adjustments, or acupuncture may provide significant pain alleviation. The main goals of these treatments are to ease muscle tension, increase circulation, and encourage relaxation.

Surgical Indications And Results

Adults with scoliosis may require surgical intervention if conservative treatment is unable to control symptoms or if the curvature of the spine becomes severe. The goals of surgery are to stabilize the spine, treat pain, and adjust curvature.

Adult-onset scoliosis can be treated surgically using a variety of techniques, such as spinal fusion, decompression, and instrumentation. In order to stabilize the spine and stop additional curvature, the vertebrae are fused together during spinal fusion using bone transplants and metal rods or screws.

In order to relieve discomfort and increase mobility, decompression procedures entail removing bone or tissue that is compressing spinal nerves. In order to straighten the spine and preserve stability, rods, screws, or other devices may be inserted during instrumentation procedures.

The degree of curvature, the patient's general health, and the particular surgical approach employed all affect how well an adult-onset scoliosis surgery goes. Many people find that surgery efficiently corrects the curvature and relieves their pain, but there are dangers involved, including the possibility of infection, blood loss, and anesthesia-related issues.

Problems With Life Quality And Coping Strategies

Having adult-onset scoliosis can cause a number of difficulties that negatively affect one's quality of life. Emotional and physical health can be negatively impacted by persistent pain, restricted movement, and bodily transformations. Nonetheless, there are coping techniques and approaches that can assist people in controlling their illness and enhancing their general quality of life.

People with scoliosis can benefit greatly from the emotional support and useful guidance that support groups and internet communities can offer. Developing relationships with people who have gone through similar things to you might help you feel less alone and more like you belong.

Sustaining a healthy lifestyle can help reduce symptoms and enhance general well-being. This includes regular exercise, eating right, and learning stress-reduction strategies. Walking, yoga, and other low-impact workouts can help increase flexibility and strengthen the muscles that support the spine.

In addition, employing supportive equipment like back braces or ergonomic seats can assist ease discomfort and lessen the strain on the spine. Seeking expert assistance from medical professionals, such as physical therapists or mental health specialists, can also be very beneficial in assisting with managing the difficulties associated with having adult-onset scoliosis.

CHAPTER SEVEN

SCOLIOSIS PREVENTION AND MAINTENANCE

Awareness Of Posture Is Crucial

For people with scoliosis, maintaining good posture is essential to preventing future issues and easing suffering.

Maintaining proper posture eases the pressure on the spine and surrounding muscles by assisting in the equal distribution of body weight. Additionally, it encourages improved spinal alignment, which may stop the curvature from getting worse.

It is imperative that you practice mindfulness throughout the day in order to build posture awareness. This entails being aware of your posture, gait, and sitting habits. Simple practices like maintaining a straight posture, releasing tension in the shoulders, and lining up the ears, shoulders, and hips can have a big impact on spinal health. In addition, feedback and direction on maintaining good alignment can be obtained by using mirrors or hiring a posture coach.

Stretching And Exercise For A Healthy Spine

In order to manage scoliosis and preserve spinal health, regular exercise, and targeted stretches can be quite beneficial. Exercises like yoga, pilates, or swimming that target the core muscles can support the spine and enhance posture. The main goals of these exercises are to increase balance, strength, and flexibility—all of which are critical for total spinal stability.

In addition to relieving stress and pain, certain stretches can also target the muscles that surround the spine.

Exercises that stretch the spine and increase flexibility in the shoulders, hips, and back can help release tension and increase the range of motion. You may prevent stiffness and soreness in your spine by including simple twists, bends, and extension movements in your everyday routine.

Ergonomic Guidelines For Typical Tasks

People with scoliosis may experience less discomfort and less strain on their spines by incorporating ergonomic principles into their regular routines.

Simple changes to your surroundings and posture can have a major impact, whether you're at work, at home, or engaging in leisure activities.

Maintaining a neutral spine position and selecting a chair with adequate lumbar support when seated will help reduce back discomfort and slouching.

In addition to ensuring correct alignment, raising or lowering desks, displays, and keyboards can help improve posture and lessen tiredness.

When lifting, hauling, or doing repeated chores, it's crucial to take posture and body mechanics into account in addition to seating ergonomics.

Injuries can be avoided and spinal strain can be reduced by using safe lifting techniques, avoiding twisting motions, and taking regular breaks to stretch and relax.

Dietary Aspects Of Bone Health

Maintaining bone health is mostly dependent on diet, which is especially crucial for those who have scoliosis.

Bone strength and density can be supported by eating a balanced diet high in calcium, magnesium, vitamin D, and other vital nutrients.

Building and maintaining strong bones require calcium, and bone remodeling and calcium absorption are facilitated by vitamin D.

You can make sure you're getting enough of these nutrients by including dairy products, leafy greens, nuts, seeds, and fortified foods in your diet.

Magnesium, along with calcium and vitamin D, is essential for muscular contraction and bone metabolism.

Good sources of magnesium include leafy greens, nuts, seeds, and whole grains; these foods should be a part of a balanced diet.

Frequent Exams And Preventive Actions

People with scoliosis must see medical professionals on a regular basis to track the condition's development and swiftly address any concerns.

Physical therapists and orthopedic professionals, among others, are qualified to evaluate spinal curvature, track changes over time, and suggest suitable interventions.

Preventive strategies can assist manage scoliosis and prevent problems, in addition to routine medical checkups. These methods include wearing supportive braces, engaging in focused physical therapy programs, and avoiding activities that increase symptoms.

People with scoliosis can reduce discomfort, preserve mobility, and improve the overall quality of life by being proactive about spine health and implementing preventive measures in daily life.

CHAPTER EIGHT

A FAQ AND A COMMON ASK:

Could Scoliosis Be Avoided?

It is challenging to completely prevent scoliosis since the majority of instances occur during adolescent growth spurts when bones are expanding quickly.

However, management of its advancement might be aided by early detection and intervention.

Overall spinal health can be improved by promoting excellent posture, sustaining a healthy lifestyle with frequent exercise, and making sure eating is appropriate.

Furthermore, adolescent scoliosis tests can detect problems early on and enable prompt treatment if needed.

How Might Pregnancy Be Impacted By Scoliosis?

Due to changes in posture and weight distribution, scoliosis may cause discomfort or pain during pregnancy.

Pregnancy might cause more difficulty because of the added weight and hormonal changes that can aggravate preexisting spinal curvature.

Nonetheless, many scoliosis-affected women who receive the right medical attention and supervision can have healthy pregnancies.

Working collaboratively with their healthcare providers, pregnant women with scoliosis can manage any pain or discomfort and guarantee the best possible outcome for mother and baby.

Does Age Cause Scoliosis To Worsen?

Although scoliosis usually appears during adolescence, in certain situations, it can worsen or advance with age.

The degree of curvature, overall spinal health, and heredity are some of the factors that can affect how scoliosis develops over time.

The curvature of the spine can also be affected by changes in muscle strength and bone density as people age.

In order to assess any changes in scoliosis and determine the best course of action, which may involve bracing, surgery, or physical therapy, depending on the severity, regular monitoring by a healthcare practitioner is required.

Are There Any Scoliosis Natural Therapies Available?

While there are no all-natural treatments for scoliosis, some hobbies and lifestyle choices may help manage symptoms and enhance spinal health. Improved posture and relief from scoliosis-related discomfort can be achieved with the aid of yoga, pilates, and targeted workouts that focus on strengthening and stretching the core. Overall spinal health can also be influenced by keeping a healthy weight, adopting proper posture, and avoiding activities that put stress on the spine. To make sure it's safe and appropriate for their particular condition, it's crucial to speak with a healthcare provider before beginning any new fitness program, especially for those who have scoliosis.

What recent developments exist in the management of scoliosis?

Treatment choices for scoliosis patients are increasing as a result of ongoing advancements in the field. The creation of minimally invasive surgical methods for treating spinal curvature is one noteworthy breakthrough. Compared to open operations, these techniques usually include fewer incisions, less blood loss, and quicker recovery periods. Additionally, 3D-printed braces, which are tailored to each patient's specific anatomy, are an example of how advances in bracing technology have made traditional braces less uncomfortable and more effective. Future developments in treating scoliosis may be possible thanks to research into tissue engineering and genetic medicines, which may provide some patients with surgical alternatives.

To ascertain the best course of action depending on unique circumstances like age, the degree of curvature, and general health, it is imperative to speak with a healthcare provider.

www.ingramcontent.com/pod-product-compliance
Lightning Source LLC
Chambersburg PA
CBHW071841210526
45479CB00001B/237